AMYLOIDOSIS

A Comprehensive Guide to The Amyloidosis Handbook: From Symptoms to Solutions

CARL JUAN

Table of Contents

Introductory

Rare and complicated, amyloidosis is defined by the buildup of amyloid proteins in cells, tissues, and organs. In amyloidosis, usually soluble amyloid proteins misfold and clump to produce insoluble fibrils that can accumulate in different areas of the body. This accumulation of amyloid fibrils can alter normal tissue structure and function, resulting to a wide range of symptoms and potentially causing organ damage.

• Different forms of amyloidosis are linked to the accumulation of different proteins. Amyloidosis comes in a variety of forms, including:

• Primary amyloidosis (also known as AL amyloidosis) is characterized by the buildup of aberrant immunoglobulin light chains (amyloidogenic light chains) and is frequently linked to diseases of the plasma cells, such as multiple myeloma.

• The amyloid A protein, an acute-phase reactant created in response to persistent inflammation or infection, has been related to the development of this form of secondary amyloidosis.

- Amyloidosis of transthyretin (ATTR) occurs when transthyretin (TTR) protein misfolds and accumulates in the body. ATTR amyloidosis can be either inherited (familial) or acquired (wild-type).

- Amyloid-beta (A) amyloidosis is most commonly linked to Alzheimer's disease due to the accumulation of amyloid-beta (A) protein in the brain.

- Individuals with ESRD who have been on dialysis for an extended period of time can develop amyloidosis. The protein beta-2 macroglobulin tends to build up in this condition.

Depending on the nature and location of the amyloid deposits, the specific symptoms and organ involvement in amyloidosis can vary. Common symptoms may include weariness, weight loss, edema (swelling), organ malfunction, and neuropathy (nerve damage). Management techniques for amyloidosis may include chemotherapy, organ transplantation, or drugs that target the underlying illness processes, and diagnosis is often a team effort.

As a group of disorders, amyloidosis spans a wide spectrum of conditions, each of which requires a unique approach to diagnosis, treatment, and care.

CHAPTER ONE
Amyloidosis: What You Need to Know

Because it can lead to so many different health issues, amyloidosis is a major medical concern. It's crucial for a number of reasons:

• Disruption of Normal Structure and Function of Organs: Amyloidosis can cause the buildup of amyloid proteins in different tissues and organs. Without treatment, this might cause irreversible organ damage and ultimately organ failure. The organs affected by amyloidosis range from heart to kidneys to liver to nerves and beyond.

• Amyloidosis is difficult to diagnose since its symptoms might be vague and similar to those of other disorders. Depending on which organs are affected, the range of symptoms can be rather broad, but common ones include fatigue, weight loss, edema, neuropathy, and heart difficulties. Because of this variety, diagnoses may be missed or given incorrectly.

• In some cases, amyloidosis can be traced back to an underlying disease. Examples include the correlation between AA amyloidosis and chronic inflammatory diseases and the association between AL amyloidosis and multiple myeloma. The underlying disease must be treated in such circumstances.

• Amyloidosis can have a devastating effect on many generations of a family if it is a hereditary kind, such as ATTR amyloidosis. Managing these conditions requires early diagnosis and genetic counseling.

• The prognosis for amyloidosis varies according to a number of factors, such as the specific kind and the degree of organ involvement. The outlook is better for some forms than others. Combinations of chemotherapy, organ transplantation, and anti-amyloid medicines are commonly used for treatment. Complex conditions may necessitate individualized treatment plans.

• Due of amyloidosis' importance in the context of numerous disorders, research and medication development are ongoing to better understand the condition and improve treatment options. This encompasses experimental treatments, clinical studies, and cutting-edge strategies for eliminating amyloid deposits.

• Amyloidosis can have a devastating effect on a person's quality of life. Disability and a reduction in one's capacity to carry out regular tasks may result from symptoms such as neuropathy and organ dysfunction. Patients with amyloidosis can benefit greatly from effective treatment that extends their lifespan.

The potential for severe health problems, the difficulty in diagnosis and treatment, the link with other diseases, and the impact on patients and their families all contribute to amyloidosis' relevance. Medical practitioners and researchers continue to strive towards increasing the understanding and management of this illness. Improving outcomes and quality of life for people with amyloidosis requires prompt diagnosis and treatment.

The Origins of Amyloid

The biological process of amyloid production involves the aggregation of soluble proteins or peptides into insoluble fibrils or plaques. These fibrils are defined by their peculiar structure, in which the proteins form beta-sheet-rich structures and have a tendency to stack on top of one another. Amyloidosis is a set of diseases marked by this mechanism, and it is also involved in a number of neurodegenerative diseases.

Some important facts about amyloid formation are as follows:

• Proteins and peptides from a wide range of diseases are involved in amyloid formation. Amyloid-beta (A) protein clumps in Alzheimer's disease, while alpha-synuclein is involved in Parkinson's disease. Proteins including immunoglobulin light chains (AL amyloidosis) and transthyretin (ATTR amyloidosis) can misfold and aggregate, leading to amyloidosis.

• Protein Misfolding: These proteins typically have a very well-defined three-dimensional structure and role in the body. These proteins misfold, losing their usual structure, in amyloidosis and neurodegenerative disorders. Proteins with fold errors tend to clump together.

• Structure Rich in Beta-Sheets: This is a defining feature of amyloid fibrils. This indicates that the proteins or peptides implicated in amyloid formation adopt a certain shape where beta-sheet structures dominate, rendering them resistant to breakdown.

• The production of amyloid involves an aggregation mechanism that is nucleation-dependent. First, "seeds" are formed, which might then encourage the further aggregation of proteins or peptides into fibrils. Over time, this can spread and build up.

• Cellular Damage Amyloid fibril buildup can cause cellular dysfunction and morphology changes. Cellular malfunction or death may result from the accumulation of such aggregates. Neuronal damage is linked to the presence of amyloid plaques in the brain, which is especially prominent in neurodegenerative illnesses.

• Alzheimer's disease, Parkinson's disease, Huntington's disease, prion illnesses, and various kinds of amyloidosis have all been associated to amyloid production. Depending on the illness, different tissues or organs may be impacted and different proteins or peptides may be at play.

• Research and therapeutics hinge on a thorough understanding of the mechanisms behind amyloid development. As a potential therapeutic approach for many disorders, researchers are looking into ways to prevent or interrupt the process. Early detection and treatment of amyloidosis necessitate further study of the disease.

Proteins or peptides misfold and clump into insoluble fibrils, a process known as amyloid formation. Amyloid is linked to many diseases, and scientists are working hard to uncover its causes and find ways to treat or prevent them.

CHAPTER TWO
Presentation in the Clinic

In the context of a medical examination, a patient's clinical presentation is all the information the patient provides to the doctor. It is a crucial element of the diagnostic process that helps healthcare professionals analyze a patient's health status, establish the underlying medical condition, and arrange suitable therapy or further examination. Depending on the patient, the underlying medical condition, and the healthcare facility, the clinical presentation may or may not include the following:

• Patient provides details on their own and their family's medical history, including conditions treated, procedures performed, drugs taken, allergic reactions experienced, and other lifestyle factors such as smoking, diet, and physical activity. Potential contributors to their present health problems and risk factors can be determined with this data.

• A patient's symptoms may include pain, exhaustion, nausea, dizziness, or any other physical or mental sensations the patient reports feeling. Patients report on the location, kind, duration, and severity of their symptoms, as well as any contributing or mitigating circumstances.

• During a patient's physical examination, a doctor or nurse will make a number of objective observations, or "signs." Vital signs include blood pressure, heart rate, and temperature; physical findings include edema, rashes, abnormal heart sounds, and neurological impairments; and laboratory results include blood, urine, and saliva samples.

• The health care provider's ability to evaluate the patient's condition as a whole depends on the results of a complete physical examination. In order to detect abnormalities, it may be necessary to visually examine, palpate (feel), percuss (touch), and auscultate (listen) various parts of the body.

• Imaging studies (such as X-rays, CT scans, and MRIs), as well as other diagnostic procedures, such as blood and urine testing, provide further information. The results of these examinations can be used to corroborate or disprove hypotheses about the patient's health.

• Even if a patient is not complaining of any symptoms related to a particular organ system, doctors will nevertheless ask about it as part of a comprehensive review of the patient's overall health. This can assist discover any problems or conditions that the patient may not have mentioned.

• A healthcare clinician will compile a list of potential diagnoses, or a differential diagnosis, based on the information gathered. This entails thinking about potential medical issues that could cause the patient's signs and symptoms.

- Healthcare personnel assess the situation and come up with a plan for therapy or management based on the patient's clinical presentation, medical history, and diagnostic findings. This may involve prescription drugs, advocating lifestyle modifications, ordering further tests, or referring the patient to experts.

In order to make an accurate diagnosis, a thorough understanding of the patient's clinical presentation is essential. It's useful for figuring out what treatment and follow-up are needed. Effective medical treatment requires a combination of clinical expertise and diagnostic tools with complete and accurate patient reporting.

Biology of Amyloidosis

Some types of amyloidosis, such as hereditary or familial amyloidosis, have strong genetic components. These forms of amyloidosis are brought on by inherited mutations in certain genes. Here is a quick rundown of how amyloidosis is linked to genetics:

• Amyloidosis that runs in families is called hereditary amyloidosis, and it is caused by changes in one or more genes. Hereditary amyloidosis has been linked to two well-studied genes, including:

- **Transthyretin (TTR) Gene:** Transthyretin amyloidosis (or ATTR amyloidosis) is caused by mutations in the TTR gene. ATTR amyloidosis comes in several forms, including the variant (ATTRv) and the mutant (ATTRm) forms. Amyloid deposits develop in several organs, including the brain, heart, and intestines, when a mutated form of the transthyretin protein is produced.

Amyloid deposits in the kidneys are a symptom of hereditary renal amyloidosis, which is caused by mutations in the fibrinogen alpha chain (AFib) gene.

• Hereditary amyloidosis follows an autosomal dominant pattern of inheritance. This indicates that each child of a parent who contains a disease-causing mutation has a 50% chance of inheriting the mutation and developing the disease. These mutations are potentially heritable, which means they can cause disease in future generations.

• **Genetic Testing**: Genetic testing can uncover mutations in the TTR and AFib genes, as well as other genes implicated with hereditary amyloidosis. Amyloidosis risk assessment testing is essential for anyone with a family history of the disease. Early detection and treatment may potentially benefit from this.

• Individuals with a family history of hereditary amyloidosis may benefit from genetic counseling. Family planning and genetic testing choices can be discussed with genetic counselors, as can the inheritance pattern and the danger of passing the mutation on to future generations.

• The therapy of hereditary amyloidosis may be affected by our understanding of its genetic origin. Some new treatments aim to correct the underlying genetic abnormalities that cause disease. Treatments for diseases like ATTR amyloidosis focus on preventing the aberrant transthyretin protein from being produced or stabilizing existing levels of the protein.

• Not all cases of amyloidosis can be traced back to a family history of the disease. The majority of people who develop amyloidosis do not have a predisposing genetic mutation. Caused by aging, chronic inflammation, or other underlying medical issues.

Accurate diagnosis, risk assessment, and individualized treatment techniques depend on a firm grasp of amyloidosis's genetic foundations. Genetic testing and counseling can be important tools for individuals and families at risk of hereditary amyloidosis, helping them make educated decisions about their health and well-being.

CHAPTER TWO
Predisposing Genes

Genetic risk factors are inherited characteristics that raise an individual's vulnerability to a disease or health problem. A person's vulnerability to disease is largely determined by their genetic makeup, which can be passed down from their parents. To better understand genetic risk factors, consider the following:

1. Genetic differences: Certain differences in an individual's DNA are often linked to particular genetic risk factors. Gene function can be altered by these changes, potentially making a person more susceptible to a disease.

2. Risk factors can run in a family and be passed down from generation to generation. This means that a person's risk for a disease can be passed down through their genes if one or both of their parents carry the genetic variant linked to that disease.

3.Many common diseases have complicated genetic risk factors, including heart disease, diabetes, cancer, and some neurological problems. Many different genes play a role in increasing the likelihood of developing certain diseases.

4. Some illnesses, known as monogenic disorders, stem from a single mutation in a single gene. In certain instances, the ailment can be traced back to a specific mutation. Diseases like CF, Sickle Cell Anemia, and Huntington's are just a few examples.

5. Polygenic Diseases: Most diseases, however, are polygenic, meaning they result from the combined actions of numerous genes. Many genes contribute to the risk of polygenic disorders, however each gene variation only accounts for a small percentage of the overall risk.

6. Researchers employ GWASs to find potential genetic risk factors for complicated diseases. These studies look for common genetic variants related with an illness by analyzing the genomes of large groups of people. These variants may increase susceptibility, but they are by no means a surefire predictor of disease.

7. Variables in the Environment: It's not uncommon for environmental risk variables to interact with genetic risk factors. When combined with other risk factors, such as nutrition, lifestyle, or chemical exposure, certain genetic variants may increase disease vulnerability.

8. Genetic testing allows people to learn about their familial propensity for developing diseases. Breast cancer runs in families, therefore someone with a strong family history of the disease might get tested for BRCA1 and BRCA2 mutations to see if they have an elevated risk of developing breast and ovarian cancer.

9. Treatments and interventions in personalized medicine are increasingly based on a patient's genetic profile, which is determined by analyzing their DNA. Health care plans that take this into account have the potential to be more efficient and specific.

It's crucial to recognize that genetic risk factors are simply one component of disease risk. Major factors in determining whether an individual will develop a particular condition include one's way of life, one's surroundings, and random chance. Disease risk and healthcare decisions should take genetic risk factors into account alongside other risk factors.

Amyloid proteins accumulate abnormally in many different tissues and organs in people with hereditary amyloidosis, a group of extremely rare genetic illnesses. Inherited amyloidosis is caused by mutations in a single gene that can be passed down through families. Amyloid protein implicated in hereditary amyloidosis might vary depending on the precise genetic mutation that causes the disease. ATTR amyloidosis and hereditary Apo lipoprotein A1 amyloidosis are the two most common kinds of inherited amyloidosis. The following is a brief summary of these factors:

1. Amyloidosis Transthyretin Receptor Mutated (ATTR):

• Mutations in the TTR (transthyretin) gene are the genetic basis for ATTR amyloidosis. Amyloidosis has been linked to over a hundred different mutations in this particular gene.

• **Amyloid Protein:** Mutations in the TTR gene lead to the synthesis of aberrant transthyretin protein, which creates amyloid deposits. Tissues outside of the central nervous system, heart, and gut can also acquire these deposits.

The autosomal dominantly inherited ATTRv (Variant) variant of amyloidosis causes a wide variety of symptoms due to its variable organ involvement.

Autosomal recessive inheritance is normal for ATTRm (Mutant) amyloidosis, which occurs when mutations occur in both copies of the TTR gene. Familial amyloid polyneuropathy (FAP) is a disorder that mostly affects the nerves.

## 2.	Apo	lipoprotein	A1 amyloidosis is a genetic disorder.

• Mutations in the APOA1 gene, which codes for Apo lipoprotein A1, are the root cause of hereditary apolipoprotein A1 amyloidosis. The circulation of cholesterol depends on this protein's presence.

• Amyloid Protein: Abnormal Apo lipoprotein A1 is produced due to APOA1 gene mutations, and this abnormal protein primarily accumulates in the kidneys to generate amyloid deposits.

o Renal Involvement: Amyloidosis of this type is associated with proteinuria (abnormally high levels of protein in the urine) and, ultimately, kidney failure.

Hereditary amyloidosis: the essentials

• These disorders are inherited in a Mendelian fashion, with variable inheritance patterns depending on the precise mutation and gene involved.

• The kind of hereditary amyloidosis and the organs affected can have a significant impact on the symptoms and course of the disease.

• Diagnosing hereditary amyloidosis and pinpointing the causal mutation requires genetic testing. This can aid in the early diagnosis of affected individuals and the management of their families.

• Stabilizing the aberrant protein, decreasing its synthesis, or organ transplantation are all potential treatments for hereditary amyloidosis, depending on the patient's state and the affected organs.

Complex and often debilitating, hereditary amyloidosis calls for expert medical attention. People with amyloidosis should collaborate closely with medical professionals trained to treat the condition.

Genetic testing is a type of medical analysis used to detect and characterize particular changes in an individual's DNA. There are a number of ways in which the results of these tests can improve one's health and one's own decision-making. Here are a few essential facts concerning genetic analysis:

1. Genetic Testing's Ultimate Goals:

• Genetic testing aids in the diagnosis of hereditary diseases and disorders. The existence or absence of disease-causing mutations in a person's DNA can be determined.

Hereditary malignancies, cardiovascular diseases, and neurological disorders are only few of the diseases for which genetic testing can predict an individual's risk.

• Carrier Screening: This is a method for identifying people who may pass on harmful genetic mutations to their offspring through a process called prenatal testing.

• **Pharmacogenomics**: Individuals' responses to drugs can be tailored by genetic testing that reveals how these factors interact.

• **Ancestry and Genealogy**: Some genetic tests can reveal information on an individual's ancestry and genetic heritage.

2. Genealogical Analysis:

The purpose of diagnostic testing is to make or confirm a medical diagnosis.

- **Predictive Testing:** Determines future susceptibility to disease by locating causal genetic mutations.

- **Carrier Testing:** Detects people who harbor a disease-causing genetic mutation but who don't yet exhibit any symptoms; useful for family planning.

To determine how an individual's genetic composition impacts their response to specific medications, pharmacogenomic testing is performed.

- **Ancestry Testing:** Discovering one's genetic roots and learning about one's family tree.

3. The Genetic Counseling process typically includes genetic testing. Genetic counselors assist patients process their test results, cope with their emotions, and make educated decisions regarding their health and family planning.

4. Ethical and Privacy Considerations Ethical and privacy considerations arise while doing genetic testing. People need to know who will have access to their genetic data and how that data will be secured. The psychological and emotional effects of receiving test findings should not be ignored.

5. Individuals often give informed permission for genetic testing before undergoing the procedure, indicating that they understand the need for the test, the potential outcomes, and the intended use of the results.

6. Genetic Testing and Insurance: In some countries, genetic test findings may effect insurance coverage. Knowing the insurance and legal consequences of genetic testing in your area is crucial.

7. Many countries have laws in place to govern genetic testing to guarantee the validity and accuracy of the results. The specifics of this rule may change based on the nature of the test and the jurisdiction in which it is administered.

8. Genetic testing can be expensive depending on factors like the type of test ordered, the level of analysis required, and the patient's insurance coverage. Ancestry and health-related testing may be obtained at low cost from some direct-to-consumer genetic testing companies.

Health professionals, prospective parents, and individuals all stand to benefit from the knowledge gained through genetic testing. It's a potent resource that, in the right hands, may help people make educated choices about their health and genetics.

Amyloidosis is a collection of disorders characterized by the aberrant buildup of amyloid proteins in various tissues and organs throughout the body. **Amyloidosis can be classified according to the protein that is responsible for the development of amyloid plaques. Some of the most common forms of amyloidosis are as follows:**

1. Amyloid Protein: Amyloidosis (AL) is defined by the buildup of amyloid genic light chains from aberrant immunoglobulin.

Monoclonal gammopathy, which involves aberrant plasma cells, is a common comorbidity.

• Organs Affected: AL amyloidosis can damage several organs, including the heart, kidneys, liver, and nerves.

2. Second-Stage Amyloidosis, or AA Amyloidosis:

• **Amyloid Protein:** Amyloid A protein, an acute-phase reactant generated in response to persistent inflammation or infection, accumulates and causes AA amyloidosis.

Persistent inflammatory disorders, such as rheumatoid arthritis, inflammatory bowel disease, and persistent infections, are typically co-occurring conditions.

• **Affected Organs:** Although the kidneys are the primary target of AA amyloidosis, other organs are not immune to damage.

3. Transthyretin (or ATTR) amyloidosis:

• Amyloid Protein: Transthyretin (TTR) protein misfolds and aggregates in ATTR amyloidosis.

There are two types of ATTR amyloidosis: the familial form and the wild-type variant. The wild-type version occurs in people who have never been exposed to any harmful environmental factors, while the hereditary form is linked to specific genetic mutations.

The neurological system (in the case of inherited ATTR) or the heart (in the case of wild-type ATTR) are two of the most common organs affected by ATTR amyloidosis.

4. To wit: A Amyloidosis

Amyloid- (A) amyloidosis is the most common form of amyloidosis, and it is strongly linked to Alzheimer's disease. It involves the accumulation of amyloid-beta ($A\beta$) protein in the brain.

- **Affected Organs:** Cognitive Impairment and Neurodegeneration due to Brain Damage.

5. Amyloidosis resulting from hemodialysis:

Dialysis patients with advanced renal disease often develop this kind of amyloid protein. The protein beta-2 macroglobulin tends to build up in this condition.

Dialysis-associated amyloidosis predominantly impacts the skeletal system, including the joints and bones.

6. Regional Amyloidosis:

• **Amyloid Protein:** Amyloidosis that is confined to one area of the body usually does not cause symptoms elsewhere in the body. It can arise when amyloid deposits are identified in a specific tissue or organ.

• **Affected Organs:** The presentation can vary widely depending on which organs have amyloid deposits.

7. Systemic amyloidosis in the elderly:

• Amyloid Protein: Amyloid derived from wild-type transthyretin (TTR) accumulates in the heart of elderly people with systemic amyloidosis. It has nothing to do with faulty genes.

Heart problems are the most common o Organs Affected outcome.

These are some of the main kinds of amyloidosis, each characterized by the unique amyloid protein implicated, accompanying diseases, and afflicted organs. Determining the amyloidosis subtype is crucial for effective diagnosis and treatment.

CHAPTER THREE
What is AL Amyloidosis?

Accumulation of aberrant immunoglobulin light chains (amyloidogenic light chains) in tissues and organs is the hallmark of AL amyloidosis, also known as primary amyloidosis, a rare disease. Monoclonal gammopathy, a condition of plasma cells, is commonly linked to this form of amyloidosis. To further understand AL amyloidosis, consider the following:

• The amyloid genic light chains (AL) that build up in tissues give AL amyloidosis its name. Abnormal plasma cells in the bone marrow are responsible for the production of these light chains.

- **Associated Condition:** It is typically associated with monoclonal gammopathy of unknown significance (MGUS) or multiple myeloma. Amyloid fibrils can occur in AL amyloidosis when aberrant plasma cells create an abnormally high amount of monoclonal light chains (kappa or lambda).

- Different organs can be affected by AL amyloidosis, resulting in a wide variety of symptoms and signs. The heart, kidneys, liver, nerves, and intestines are typical sites of disease manifestation. Symptoms and organ involvement may be different for different people.

• Fatigue, shortness of breath, heart-related symptoms, kidney dysfunction, neuropathy (nerve damage), gastrointestinal difficulties, and unexplained weight loss are some of the clinical manifestations of AL amyloidosis. Due to their lack of specificity, these symptoms can be difficult to identify.

• Clinical evaluation, laboratory testing (including blood and urine), biopsies (of tissue or organs), and imaging investigations all play a role in making a diagnosis. Biopsies, which look for amyloid deposits in afflicted tissues, are a crucial diagnostic tool.

• Targeting the underlying plasma cell dysfunction and decreasing generation of aberrant light chains is the major goal of treatment. Amyloidosis can be treated with stem cell transplantation, chemotherapy (similar to that used for multiple myeloma), and drugs that stabilize the amyloidogenic light chains. Symptom and complication management that is particular to an organ system is also crucial.

• Individuals with AL amyloidosis may have a positive or negative prognosis, depending on their disease stage, the type of organs affected, how well they respond to treatment, and other factors. Improving outcomes and quality of life relies on prompt diagnosis and treatment.

• Treatment for AL amyloidosis is often followed by a period of observation to gauge the patient's response to therapy and look for signs of disease recurrence.

AL amyloidosis is a difficult disease that calls for the expertise of doctors who have dealt with similar cases before. Patients with this kind of amyloidosis have a far better prognosis if they are diagnosed and treated quickly.

Alternative Treatments

Overproduction of aberrant immunoglobulin light chains leads to amyloid deposits in numerous organs, and this is why the therapy of AL amyloidosis (primary amyloidosis) often centers on addressing the underlying plasma cell problem. The goal of treating amyloidosis is to lessen the body's synthesis of the aberrant light chains and ease the disease's symptoms and effects. The particular course of treatment may change based on the patient's condition, the number of affected organs, and other considerations. AL amyloidosis can be treated with the following methods:

1. Chemotherapy:

• Chemotherapy is frequently the basis of treatment for AL amyloidosis. Its goal is to reduce the number of aberrant plasma cells in the bone marrow that generate the amyloidogenic light chains.

Common chemotherapy treatments for AL amyloidosis include cyclophosphamide and dexamethasone (CyBorD), melphalan and dexamethasone (MelD), cyclophosphamide plus lenalidomide (LenDex), and bortezomib-based combinations.

2. Treatment Using Donated Stem Cells:

• Patients with AL amyloidosis who are candidates for high-dose chemotherapy followed by autologous stem cell transplantation (ASCT) should explore this option. The purpose of ASCT is to transplant healthy plasma cells in place of the aberrant ones.

- Stem cell transplantation is normally reserved for patients who are regarded good candidates based on their age, overall health, and level of organ involvement.

3. Medication for Amyloid genic Protein Stabilization:

- Some kinds of ATTR amyloidosis, not AL amyloidosis, may benefit from the stabilization of amyloidogenic transthyretin (TTR) proteins with the medicines tafamidis and diflunisal.

Although these drugs are not routinely used to treat AL amyloidosis, they could be an option in some patients.

4. Specific Organ Targeting:

• Organ-specific therapy may be necessary, depending on the organs afflicted and the degree of organ failure. Treatment for kidney involvement, for instance, may require measures to preserve and support kidney function, while treatment for heart involvement may involve drugs to control heart failure.

5. Assistive Therapy:

• Symptoms and complications of AL amyloidosis must be managed with the help of supportive treatment. This may include drugs to manage pain, edema, and neuropathy, as well as efforts to address heart or kidney concerns.

• Patients may also receive nutritional counseling and other forms of supportive treatment to help them stay healthy.

6. Experiments on Humans:

• Some patients with AL amyloidosis may be eligible to take part in clinical studies. Amyloidosis patients have the opportunity to participate in clinical trials for investigational treatments and therapies.

7. Keeping tabs and following up:

• Follow-up care is essential for determining whether or not a disease has returned after therapy has been administered. Amyloidosis is a chronic condition that requires constant attention from medical professionals.

The severity of symptoms, the prevalence of additional health issues, and the patient's general state of health all play a role in determining the best course of treatment. Treatment decisions are decided on an individual basis, and a multidisciplinary team of healthcare experts, including hematologists, nephrologists, and cardiologists, often collaborates to provide comprehensive care for persons with AL amyloidosis. Patients' prognoses and quality of life can be greatly improved with timely diagnosis and treatment.

CHAPTER FOUR
Inflammatory Amyloidosis

The rare condition known as AA amyloidosis is caused by the buildup of the amyloid A (AA) protein in different bodily organs and tissues. Inflammatory disorders, persistent infections, and autoimmune diseases are common risk factors for AA amyloidosis. Important details of AA amyloidosis are as follows:

1. The amyloid A (AA) protein is an acute-phase reactant produced by the liver in response to chronic inflammation or infection, and it is this protein that gives AA amyloidosis its name.

2. Chronic inflammatory disorders, such as those listed below, are typically found in patients with AA amyloidosis.

Arthritis Rheumatica

• Spondylitis (ankylosing)

Crohn's disease and ulcerative colitis are examples of inflammatory bowel disorders.

• Infections that linger for a long time, such tuberculosis and osteomyelitis

3. In AA amyloidosis, amyloid fibrils form when the liver's overproduction of the AA protein is triggered by persistent inflammation. These amyloid deposits can accumulate over time, eventually causing organ damage and dysfunction.

4. The kidneys, liver, spleen, adrenal glands, digestive tract, heart, and skin are just some of the organs that might be negatively impacted by AA amyloidosis. Symptoms and organ involvement may be different for different people.

5. Kidney dysfunction, proteinuria (excess protein in the urine), hepatomegaly (enlarged liver), splenomegaly (enlarged spleen), gastrointestinal difficulties, and cardiac issues are all possible clinical manifestations of AA amyloidosis.

6. Clinical evaluation, laboratory testing (including blood and urine), biopsies (of tissue or organs), and imaging investigations all play a role in making a diagnosis. Amyloid deposits can only be found by biopsies of damaged organs.

7. Treatment for AA amyloidosis focuses on alleviating the underlying chronic inflammatory disease that sets off the protein's overproduction. As a form of treatment,

• Disease-modifying antirheumatic medicines (DMARDs) for rheumatoid arthritis and other inflammatory diseases; these therapies reduce swelling and pain caused by the underlying disease.

• Inflammation-directed biological treatments.

• Supportive care to manage organ-specific problems.

8. Prognosis: The prognosis for patients with AA amyloidosis relies on the level of organ involvement and the efficiency of managing the underlying inflammatory illness. Improving results and limiting future organ damage require prompt diagnosis and treatment.

9. After the initial therapy, people with AA amyloidosis often need to be monitored regularly in order to evaluate their response to the medication and spot any signs of the disease returning. Consistent check-ins with medical professionals versed in amyloidosis treatment are needed.

Because of the multifaceted nature of AA amyloidosis, treatment must take into account not only the inflammatory state at its root but also the effects on affected organs. Reducing the creation of AA protein and slowing the course of amyloidosis is the key to improving outcomes in AA amyloidosis, which is why effective control of the chronic inflammatory illness is so important.

Amyloidosis involving transthyretin

Abnormal buildup of transthyretin (TTR) protein is a hallmark of ATTR amyloidosis, also known as transthyretin amyloidosis, a group of rare hereditary illnesses. The transfer of thyroid hormones and vitamin A requires TTR, a protein predominantly synthesized in the liver. Hereditary (familial) ATTR amyloidosis and wild-type ATTR amyloidosis are the two most common types. Important details concerning ATTR amyloidosis are as follows:

1. Amyloidosis of the ATTR gene:

• Specific mutations in the TTR gene underlie hereditary ATTR amyloidosis. These mutations lead to the creation of aberrant TTR protein, which misfolds and produces amyloid deposits.

- The mutation that causes hereditary ATTR amyloidosis is passed down through families at a 50% rate through autosomal dominant inheritance.

The organs affected by hereditary ATTR amyloidosis classify it into subtypes such as familial amyloid polyneuropathy (FAP) and familial amyloid cardiomyopathy (FAC).

2. Amyloidosis induced by the wild-type ATTR gene:

• Wild-type ATTR amyloidosis, also known as senile systemic amyloidosis, is not caused by genetic abnormalities and affects mostly elderly people.

- **Amyloid Formation:** The TTR protein misfolds and accumulates in numerous tissues, especially the heart, in wild-type ATTR amyloidosis.

The heart is a primary target of wild-type ATTR amyloidosis, which can have serious consequences.

3. Depending on the mutation and kind of ATTR amyloidosis, it can affect a variety of organs, including the heart, nerves, GI system, kidneys, and eyes.

4. Clinical Presentation: The symptoms of ATTR amyloidosis can vary widely, but they commonly include neuropathy (nerve damage), heart-related symptoms (such as heart failure), gastrointestinal abnormalities, and renal dysfunction. The organs affected determine the precise symptoms.

5. Clinical evaluation, genetic tests for TTR mutation identification, tissue biopsies for amyloid deposition detection, and imaging studies all contribute to a definitive diagnosis.

6. The goal of treating ATTR amyloidosis is to control symptoms, prevent or slow the disease's progression, and prevent consequences. Possible methods of treatment include:

• Therapies that try to stabilize TTR proteins, such as tafamidis and diflunisal.

Treatments include liver transplantation and innovative drugs like patisiran and inotersen have been effective in lowering TTR production.

• Targeted therapies for specific organs, such as heart, neurological, or other system failures.

• Care that focuses on the whole person, rather than just treating symptoms.

7. Prognosis: The prognosis for patients with ATTR amyloidosis varies depending on the specific mutation, the level of organ involvement, and the success of treatment. Better results and illness management can be achieved with prompt diagnosis and treatment.

8. Regular monitoring by medical professionals trained in the care of amyloidosis is essential for gauging therapy efficacy and spotting signs of relapse or worsening.

ATTR amyloidosis is a difficult disease that calls for expert treatment. Patients should collaborate with healthcare specialists skilled in amyloidosis management to receive the most effective therapy and care.

CHAPTER FIVE
Strategies for Diagnosis

Clinical evaluation, genetic testing, imaging studies, and tissue biopsies are all used in conjunction with one another to diagnose ATTR amyloidosis. The following are the most common methods used to identify ATTR amyloidosis:

1. Diagnosis in the Clinic:

• A thorough clinical evaluation, including a thorough medical history and physical examination, is typically the first step in the diagnostic process.

• The doctor will question about the patient's current symptoms, past medical history, and current medications.

2. Genomic Analysis:

• Diagnosing hereditary ATTR amyloidosis relies heavily on genetic testing. It can be used to detect transthyretin (TTR) gene mutations.

• Genetic testing can determine whether the patient has a TTR gene mutation and, if so, which mutation is responsible for the disease.

To distinguish between hereditary ATTR amyloidosis and wild-type

ATTR amyloidosis, which is not linked to mutations in the TTR gene, this testing is crucial.

3. Studies in Radiology:

• The presence and distribution of amyloid plaques in different organs can only be determined through imaging tests. The choice of imaging modalities may depend on the clinical presentation and the organs presumed to be impacted.

• Echocardiography, cardiac magnetic resonance imaging, and nuclear scintigraphy are all examples of cardiac imaging techniques commonly used to diagnose cardiac involvement.

• Nerve conduction investigations and imaging of peripheral nerves are two examples of neuroimaging that can be used to detect neurological involvement.

• If necessary, imaging of the digestive system, kidneys, and other afflicted organs may be carried out.

4. Biopsies of Organisms:

• Detecting amyloid deposits in tissue samples is typically necessary for a conclusive diagnosis of ATTR amyloidosis. Depending on the organ that is thought to be affected, a specific sort of biopsy may be performed.

• To confirm the presence of amyloid deposits, biopsies of organs such the heart, nerves, and kidneys are taken.

Amyloid fibrils can be seen under the microscope with the help of special staining procedures like Congo red staining.

5. Examining the Blood and Urine:

• Blood and urine tests can provide further diagnostic information. Protein electrophoresis of the patient's serum and urine can detect aberrant proteins indicative of amyloidosis.

6. Studies on Nerve Conduction:

• Nerve conduction investigations can evaluate nerve function and pinpoint anomalies related to neuropathy in circumstances where the nervous system is affected.

7. Clinical Indicators:

• Clinical factors, such as cardiac involvement and typical imaging abnormalities, can be used to diagnose wild-type ATTR amyloidosis in the absence of a TTR gene mutation.

8. Analyses Conducted by Experts:

• Cardiologists, neurologists, nephrologists, and gastroenterologists may all need to evaluate patients with ATTR amyloidosis because of the disease's potential impact on many organ systems.

Diagnosing ATTR amyloidosis can be problematic due to its wide range of clinical manifestations and the necessity for specialist testing. Having many amyloidosis specialists work together is typically necessary. The ability to intervene and manage an illness effectively depends on an early and correct diagnosis.

Alternative Treatments

Both inherited and wild-type ATTR amyloidosis require treatment aimed at stabilizing or reducing amyloid deposit development, managing symptoms, and addressing consequences. The kind of ATTR amyloidosis, the severity of organ involvement, and the patient's general health all play a role in determining the best course of treatment. ATTR amyloidosis can be treated with the following methods:

Therapies for Stabilization:

1. Tafamidis:

• Tafamidis is a drug licensed for the treatment of hereditary ATTR amyloidosis. Both tafamidis meglumine (Vyndaqel) and tafamidis (Vyndamax) are on the market.

• Transthyretin (TTR) proteins are stabilized by Tafamidis, which stops them from misfolding and forming amyloid fibrils. The disease's course may be slowed in this way.

2. Diflunisal:

In hereditary ATTR amyloidosis, diflunisal is another drug that has the potential to stabilize TTR proteins. It's a fallback for when tafamidis just won't do.

Stopping the Production of TTR:

3. Transplanting a Liver:

• Liver transplantation may be an option for treating inherited ATTR amyloidosis. The liver is the primary source of TTR protein, and replacing the liver with a healthy one can minimize the production of aberrant TTR.

People with particular mutations in the TTR gene are often candidates for a liver transplant if they meet certain requirements.

4. Treatments that Inhibit the Production of TTR:

• New therapies, such as patisiran and inotersen, aim to curb TTR protein production. Hereditary ATTR amyloidosis can be treated with these injectable medicines.

Organ-Particular Medications:

5. Care for the Heart:

• Medications to treat heart failure, reduce symptoms, and enhance heart function may be used to address ATTR amyloidosis with cardiac involvement. In extreme circumstances, a heart transplant may be considered.

6. Treatment for Neuropathy:

• In situations of neuropathy associated with ATTR amyloidosis, medicines to control pain and symptoms may be recommended. Both physical and occupational therapy have their uses.

7. Treatment of the Digestive System:

o Treatment for gastrointestinal symptoms may include dietary modifications, medicines to manage malabsorption, and supportive care for consequences.

8. Care for the Kidneys:

• If the kidneys are affected, treatment may focus on preserving and restoring renal function by addressing issues including proteinuria and hypertension.

Assistive Therapy:

9. Treatment of Symptoms:

• ATTR amyloidosis symptoms must be managed as part of treatment. This may entail providing the patient with individualized pain relief, nutritional assistance, and other forms of emotional and physical care.

10. Interprofessional Health Care:

• Cardiologists, neurologists, nephrologists, and other healthcare practitioners with expertise in amyloidosis management are typically needed to care for patients with ATTR amyloidosis.

11. Experiments on Humans:

• Participation in clinical trials may be an option for some individuals with ATTR amyloidosis. Access to investigational medicines and treatments for amyloidosis is available through clinical trials.

The kind of ATTR amyloidosis (inherited or wild-type), the existence of TTR gene mutations, the severity of organ involvement, and the patient's general health all play a role in determining the best course of treatment. In order to receive the therapy and care they need, people with ATTR amyloidosis must collaborate closely with a healthcare team knowledgeable in the management of amyloidosis. Better results and illness management can be

achieved with prompt diagnosis
and treatment.

CHAPTER SIX
Amyloidosis: A Way of Life

Amyloidosis can be difficult for patients and their loved ones to deal with, regardless of the type of amyloidosis they have. Here are some ways to deal with the illness:

1. Knowledge and Learning:

• Understanding grants agency. Find out as much as you can about the signs and symptoms, causes, and possible treatments for your particular kind of amyloidosis. If you have a firm grasp of the illness, you'll be better equipped to make educated decisions and control your symptoms.

2. Professional Health Care Providers:

• Gather a group of doctors and nurses who are familiar with amyloidosis. Depending on your condition, you may need to see a specialist such as a hematologist, cardiologist, nephrologist, or neurologist.

The most up-to-date care can be found in medical facilities that specialize in treating amyloidosis.

3. Backing Structures:

• Lean on your support network, including family, friends, and support groups. It can be reassuring and give a sense of camaraderie to talk to other people who understand what you're going through.

4. Mental Illness:

• The mental toll of caring for a chronic condition is real. If you are experiencing anxiety, depression, or any other emotional issues, it is important that you seek the help of a mental health professional or counselor.

5. Nutrition and Diet:

• Working with a qualified dietitian or nutritionist to create a food plan that meets your needs can be helpful if you have amyloidosis, which can cause problems with the digestive system. They are useful for handling specialized dietary issues including malabsorption.

6. Doing Something Physical:

• Be as active as your health permits. Strength in muscles, cardiovascular fitness, and general health are all aided by regular physical exercise. For safe and effective workout advice, check with your doctor.

7. Treatment and Medication Compliance:

• Follow your doctor's orders to the letter if you're taking medication or getting therapy. If you want to better manage your disease and increase your quality of life, following your treatment plan is essential.

8. Collaborate closely with your medical staff to address any bothersome symptoms. You may find relief from your symptoms and have a better quality of life with the help of medication, physiotherapy, and other behavioral modifications

9. Supportive and Palliative Care:

• Palliative care and hospice care can provide comfort, pain management, and emotional support for those with advanced amyloidosis or for those who may not be candidates for curative treatments.

10. Experiments on Humans:

• Think about enrolling in clinical trials if it seems like a good idea. New treatments and therapies for amyloidosis management are being investigated in clinical studies and may become available as a result.

11. Awareness and Advocacy:

Think about starting a movement to raise amyloidosis awareness. Bringing more attention to amyloidosis can benefit those living with the condition by increasing public understanding, funding for research, and community resources.

12. Help with the Law and Money:

• Think about the financial and legal ramifications, such as health insurance, disability payments, and retirement strategies. If you need help, contact a social professional or a patient advocacy group.

13. Adjustments to Your Life:

• Modify one's lifestyle as required, whether that be one's daily habits, living situation, or employment. Get help if you need to get through these changes.

Many people with amyloidosis find strategies to cope with the condition and keep their quality of life high with the help of loved ones and medical professionals. If you want your treatment plan to adapt to your changing needs, it's important to talk to your healthcare providers on a regular basis.

Conclusion

Amyloidosis refers to a spectrum of rare disorders that affects many organs and tissues and is defined by the abnormal accumulation of amyloid proteins. Amyloidosis can be classified according to the protein that is responsible for the development of amyloid plaques. Amyloidosis comes in a variety of forms, with AL amyloidosis, AA amyloidosis, ATTR amyloidosis, and others representing some of the more common ones. The symptoms, causes, and organs affected by each subtype are all distinct.

Clinical evaluation, genetic tests, imaging techniques, and tissue biopsies are often used together to diagnose amyloidosis. The ability to intervene and manage a situation effectively requires a prompt and precise diagnosis.

Different forms of amyloidosis have different treatment options, depending on the affected organs. Disease management includes a variety of techniques, including as stabilization therapies, drugs that target amyloid production, organ-specific treatments, and supportive care.

Individuals and their families affected with amyloidosis can overcome the disease's problems with the help of a strong support system, thorough education, and a dedicated medical team.

Treatments and knowledge about amyloidosis are constantly improving. Individuals with amyloidosis and their healthcare professionals should stay educated about the newest breakthroughs in diagnosis and therapy.

Ultimately, the best way to improve outcomes and quality of life for people with amyloidosis is through early diagnosis and rapid care.

Having the backing of doctors, family members, and patient advocacy groups is crucial.

THE END